Fruits and Veggies for a Stronger, Smarter You

by Michelle Blackwood

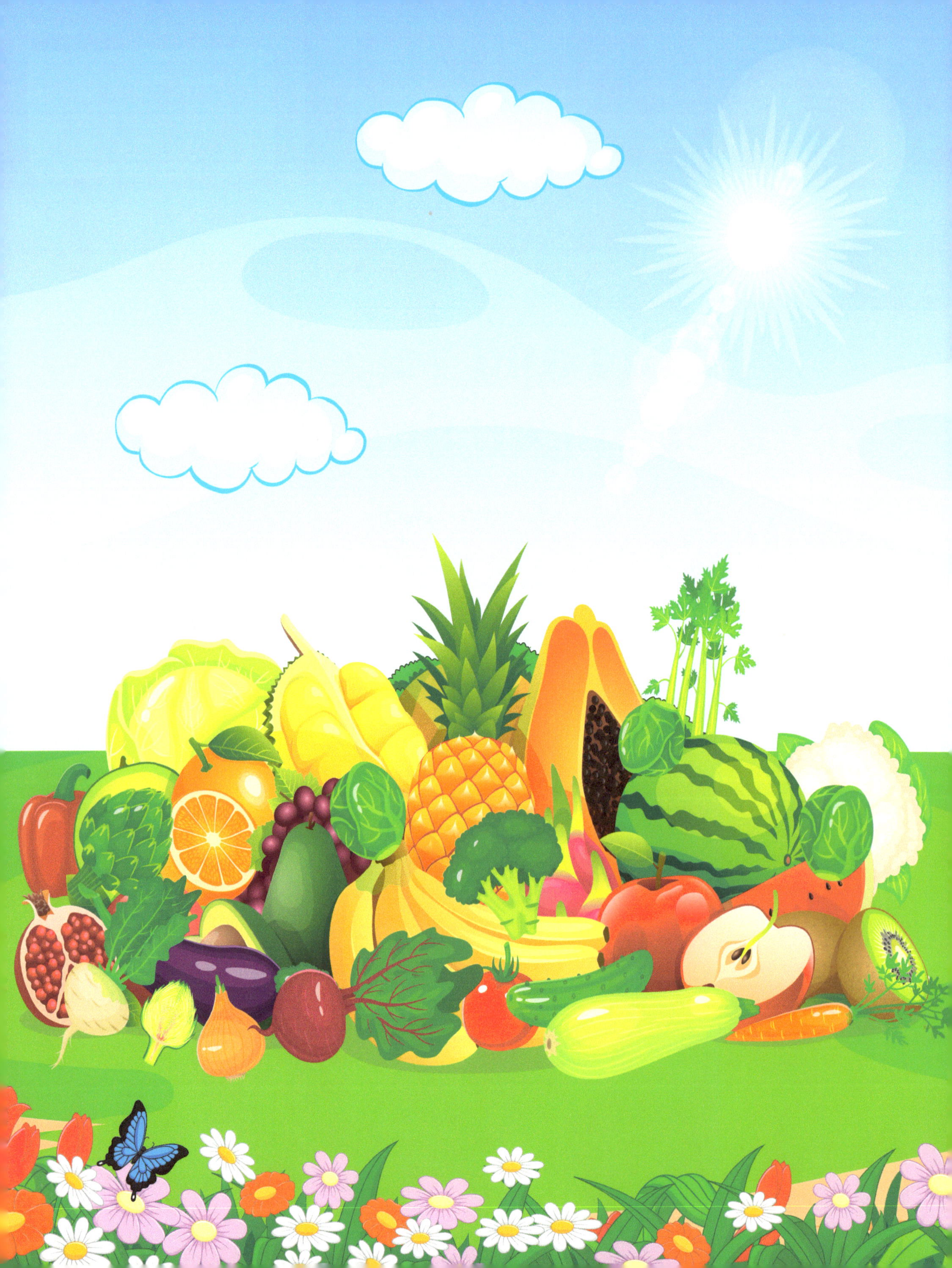

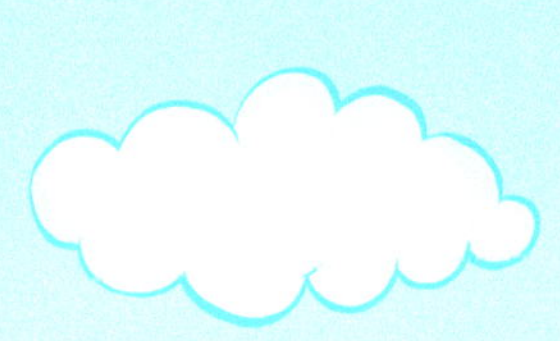

Fruits and veggies are good for you,
They help your body grow and renew.

So when you eat, make sure you choose,
Healthy foods that help you feel brand
new!

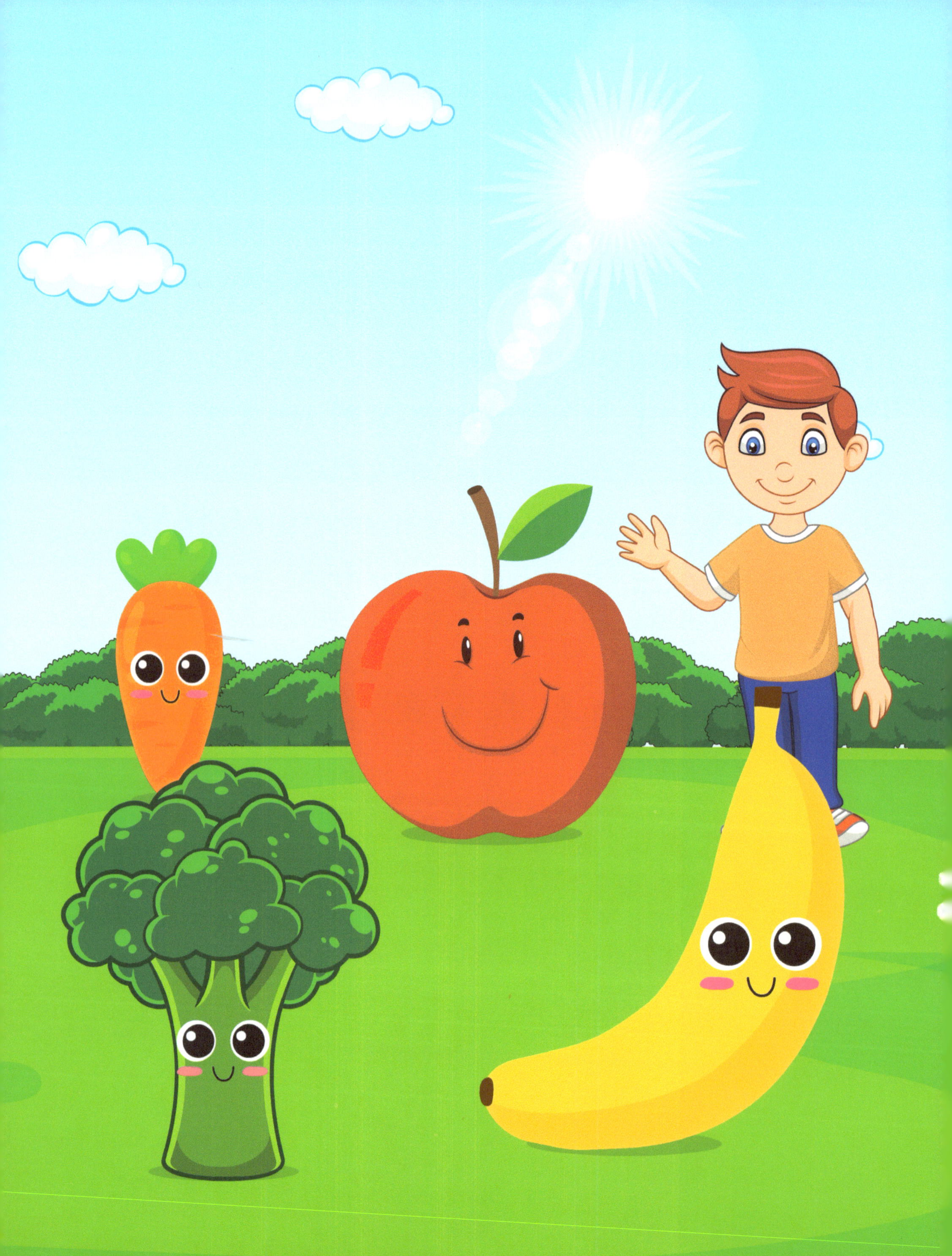

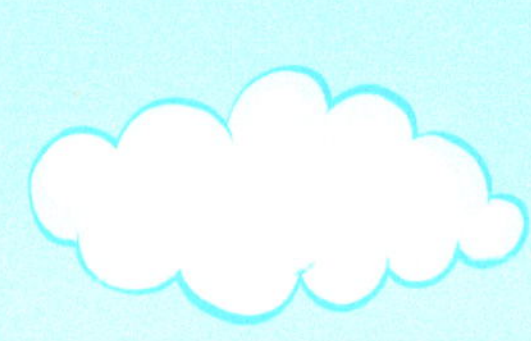

Apples make you big and strong,
Bananas help your heart sing a song!

Carrots give you superhero sight,
Broccoli keeps you feeling right!

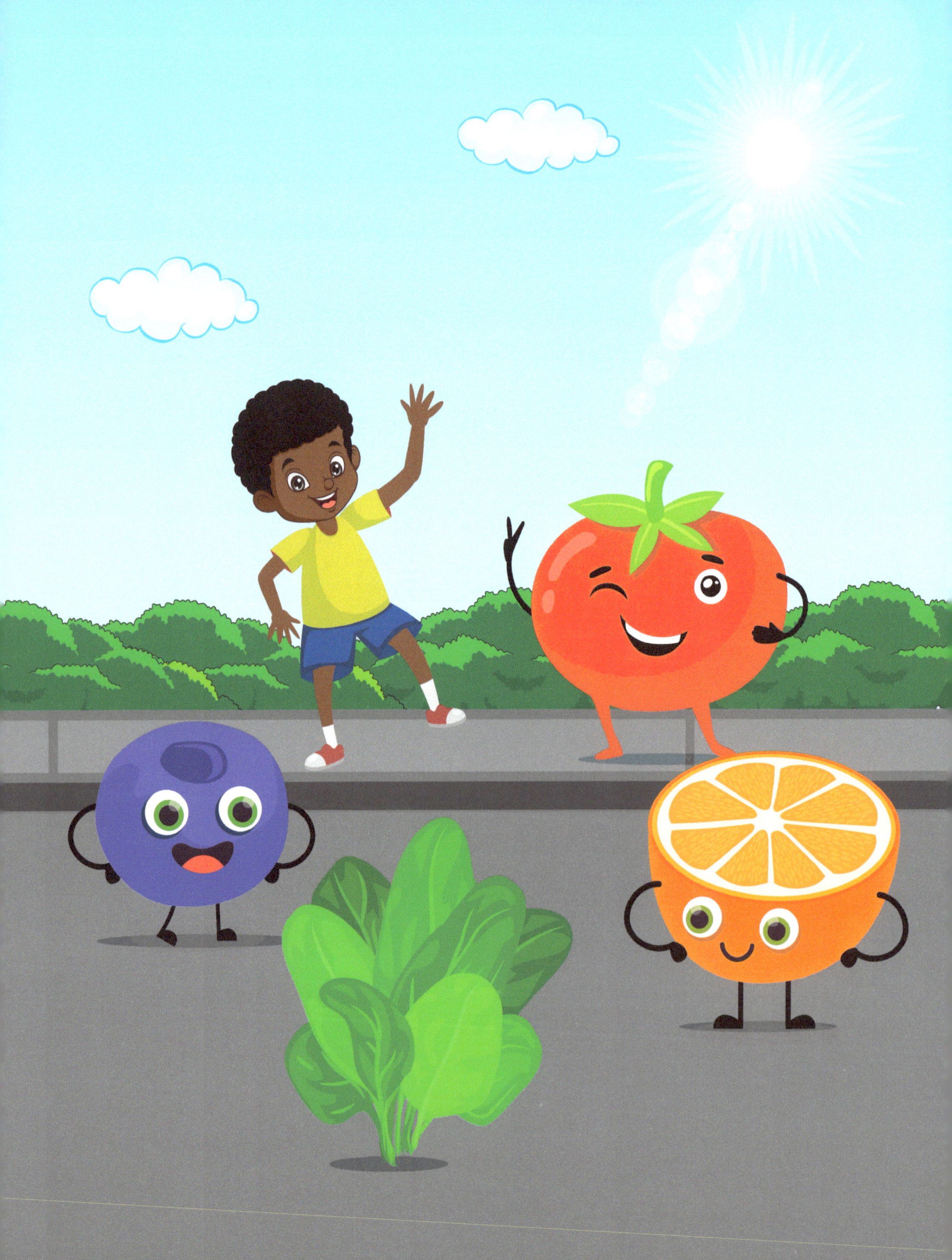

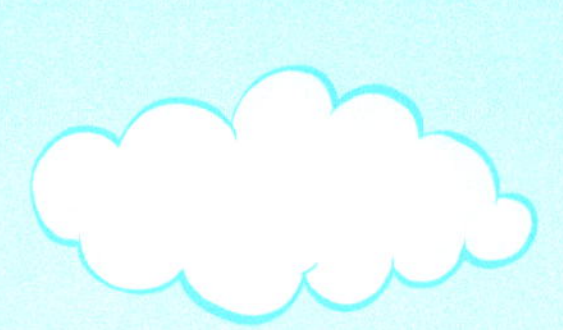

Oranges keep you feeling great, tomatoes bolster your health the whole day through. With antioxidants so strong and a vivid red hue.

Blueberries keep your mind sharp and clear, spinach helps your muscles stay in gear.

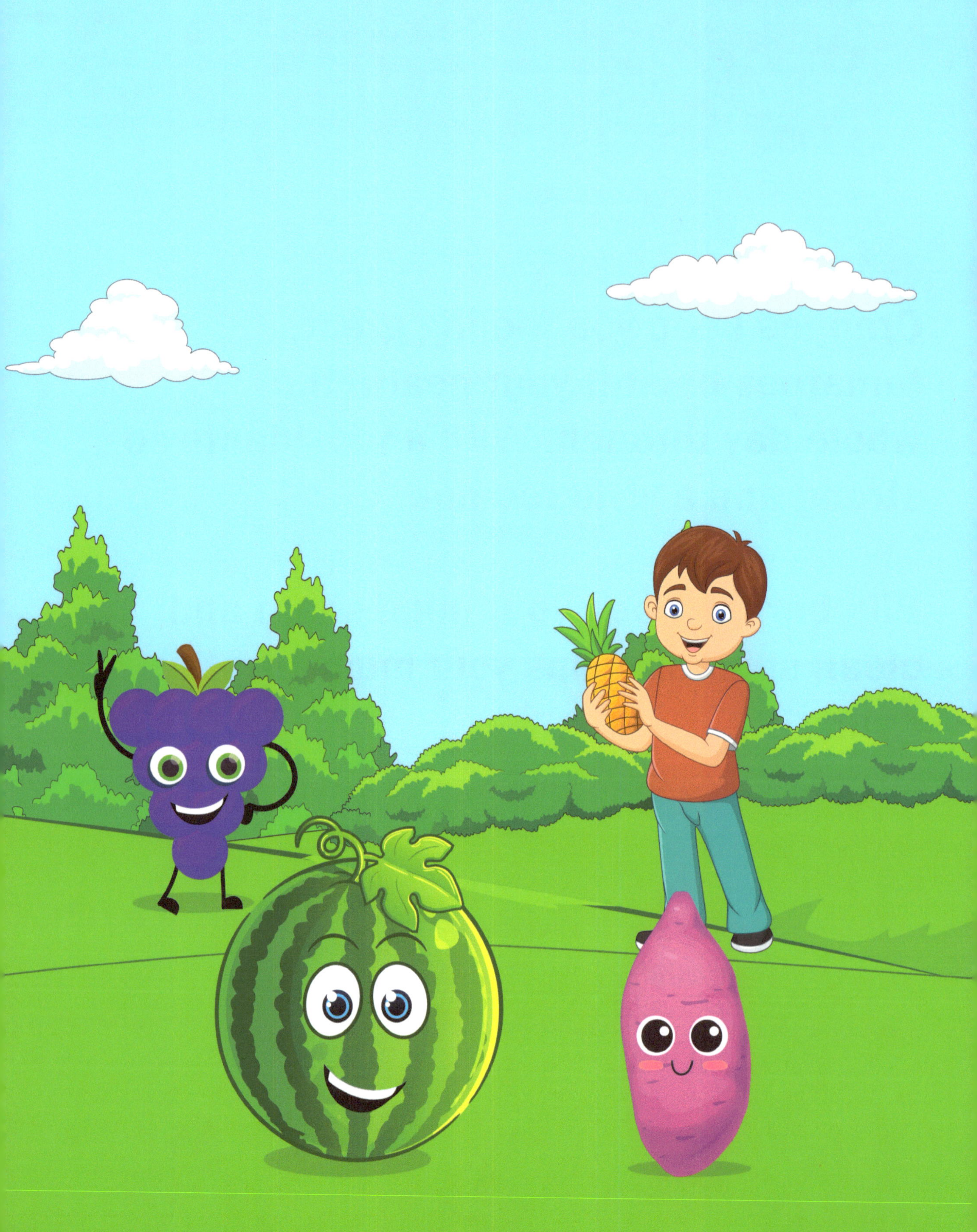

Grapes are yummy and good for you, pineapples help your digestion stay true. Watermelon keeps you hydrated and fresh.

Sweet potatoes are packed with vitamins and minerals galore, they keep our skin glowing like never before.

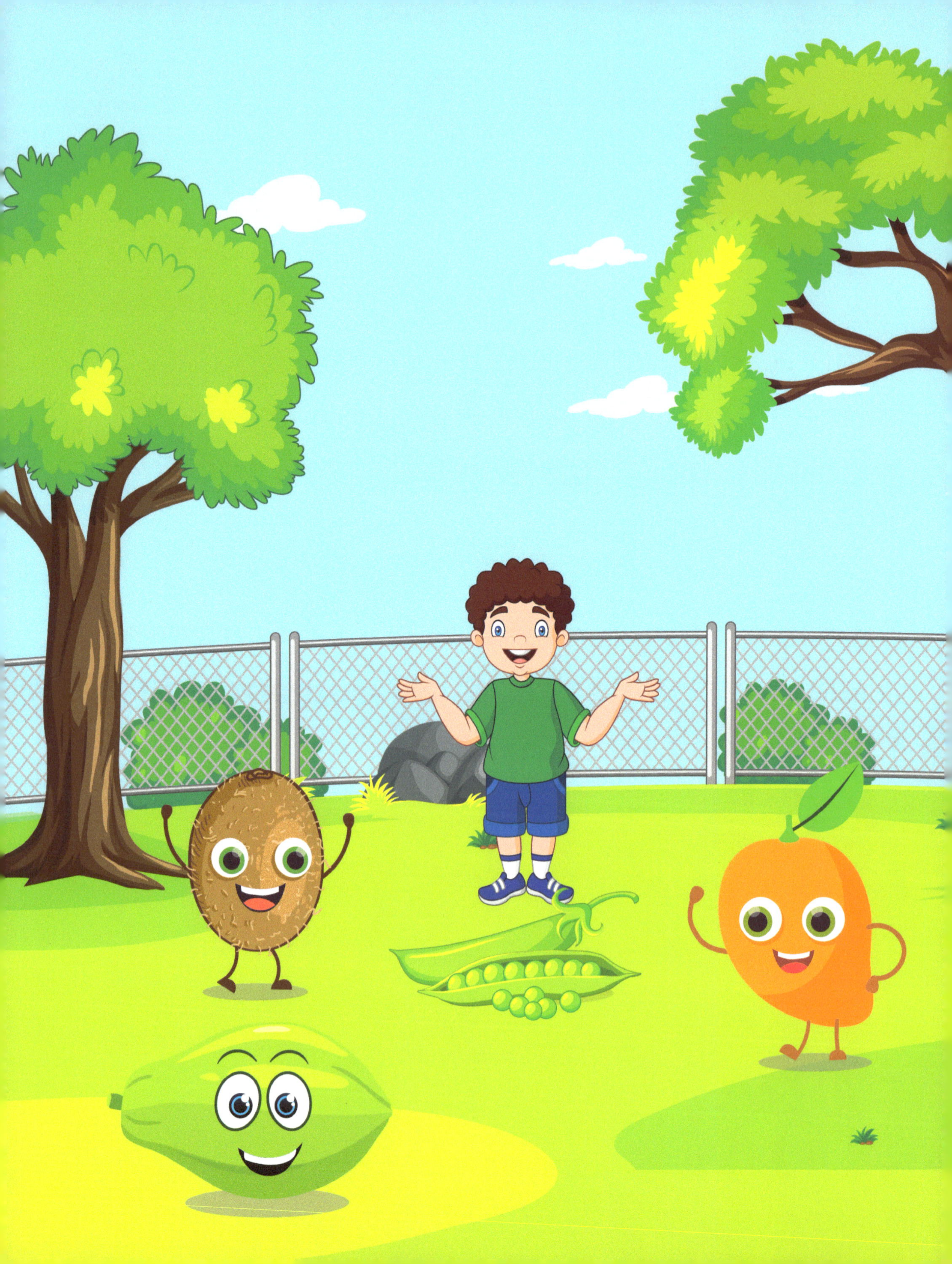

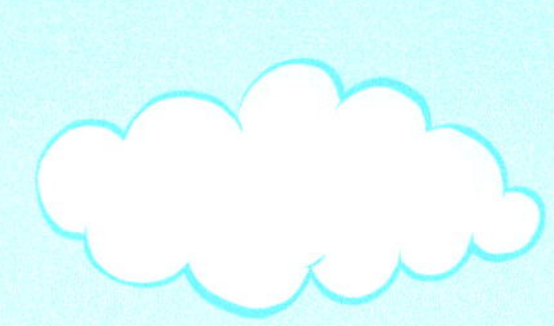

Kiwi helps keep you feeling strong,
papaya helps you digest all day long.

Mango is sweet and so much fun,
green beans help you see in the sun.

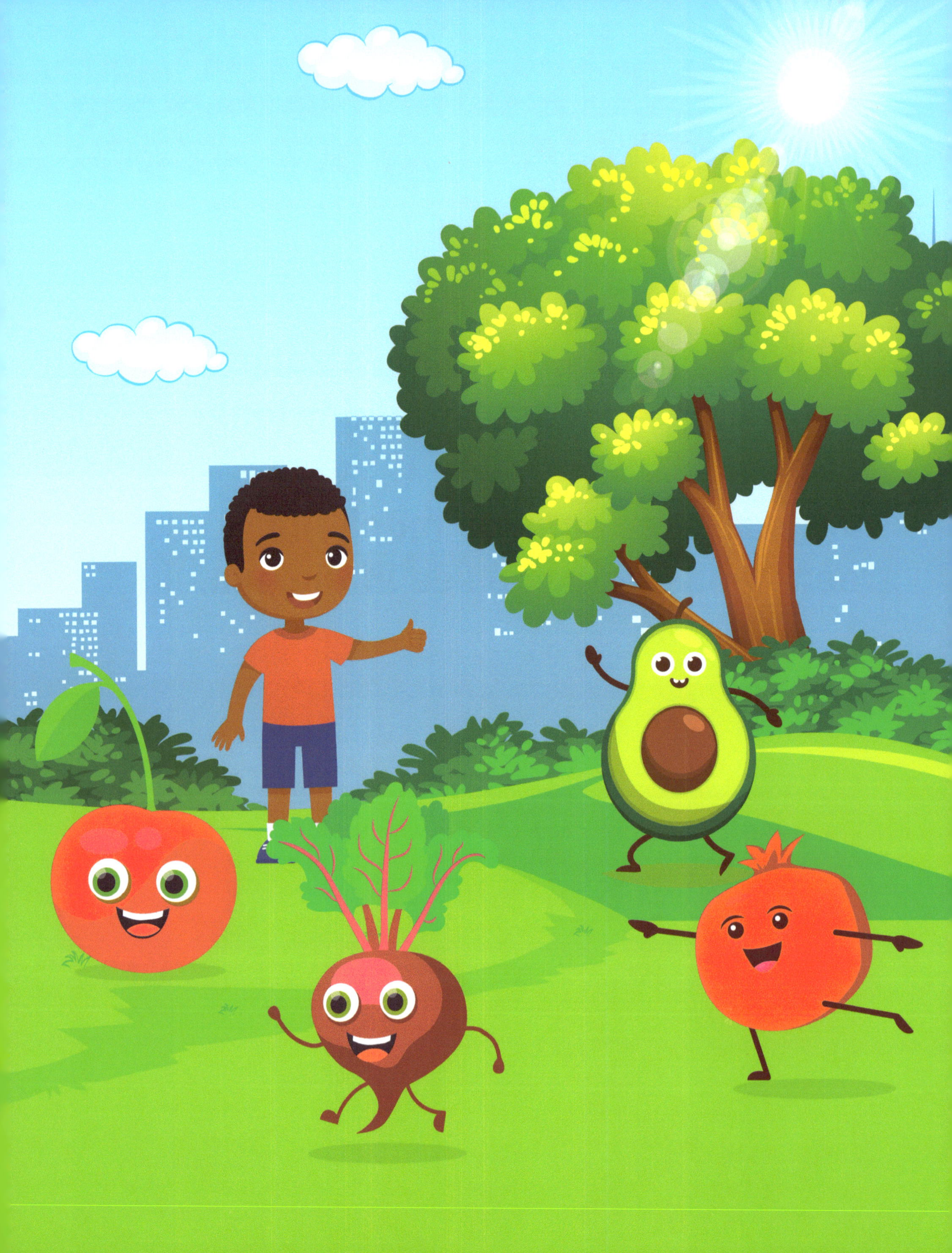

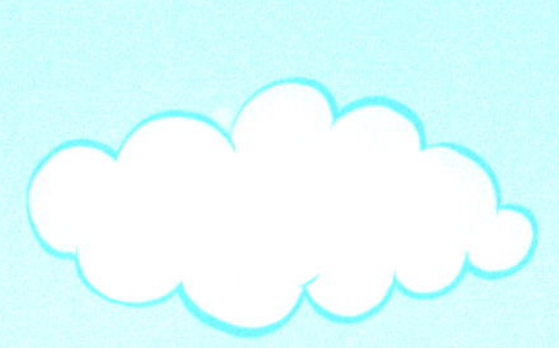

Cherries help fight off disease,
pomegranates help your blood flow with
ease.

Avocado is creamy and full of health,
beets help your body cleanse with stealth.

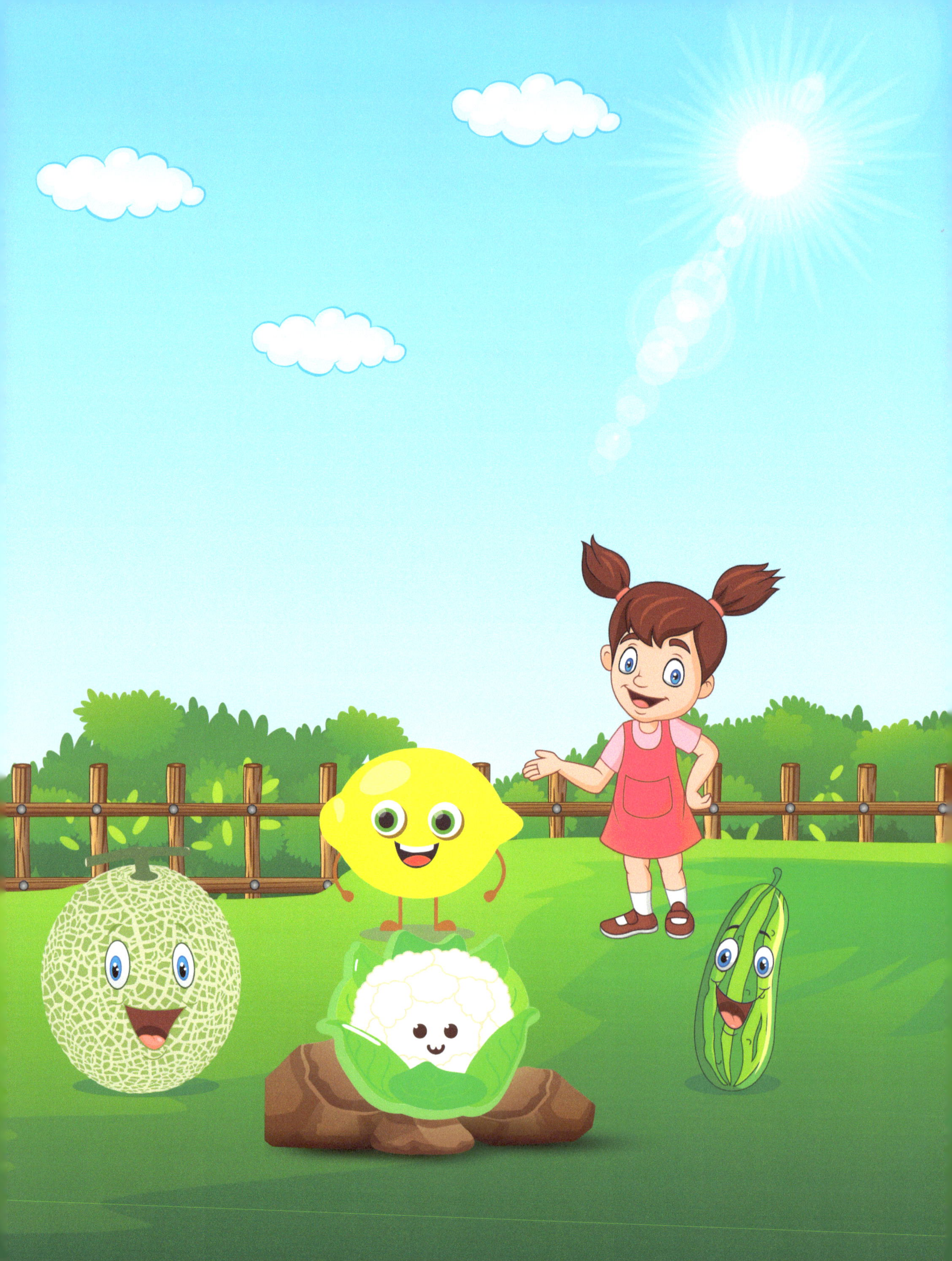

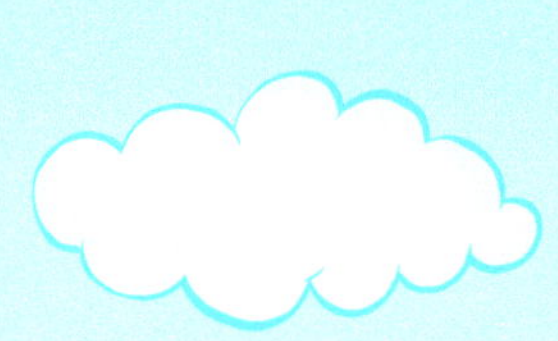

Cauliflower makes your bones tough,
cantaloupe is sweet, that's enough.

A cucumber is crunchy and cool,
lemon juice makes a tasty drink, it's no
fool.

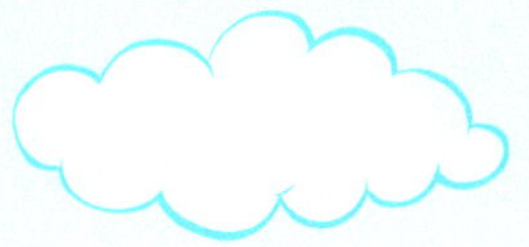

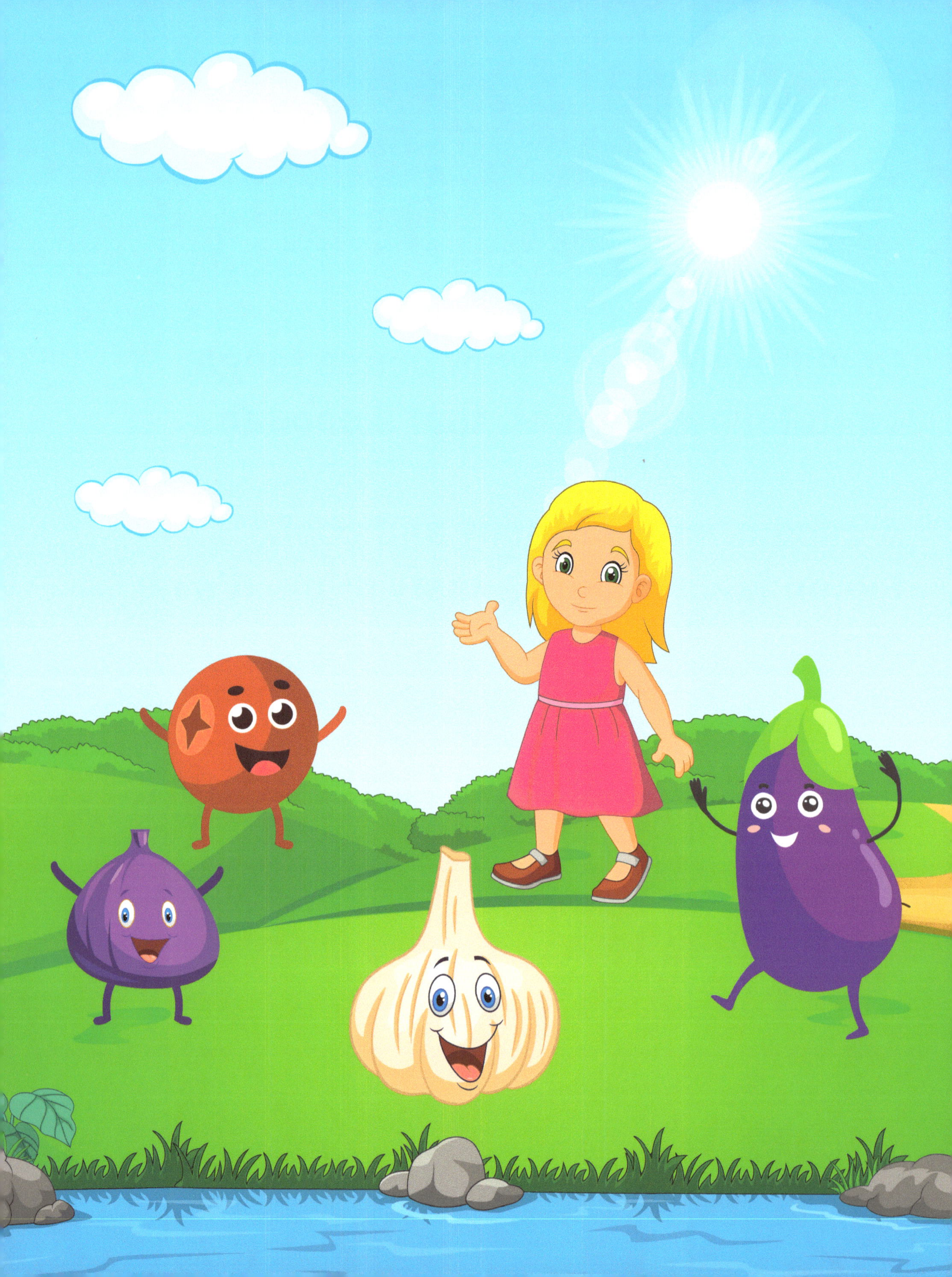

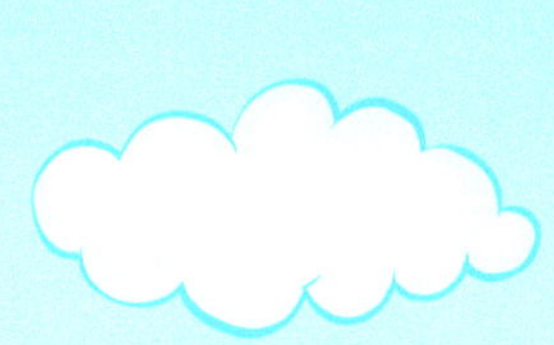

Cranberries are tart and good for you,
eggplant helps your blood sugar stay true.

Figs are sweet and full of delight,
garlic helps your cholesterol take flight.

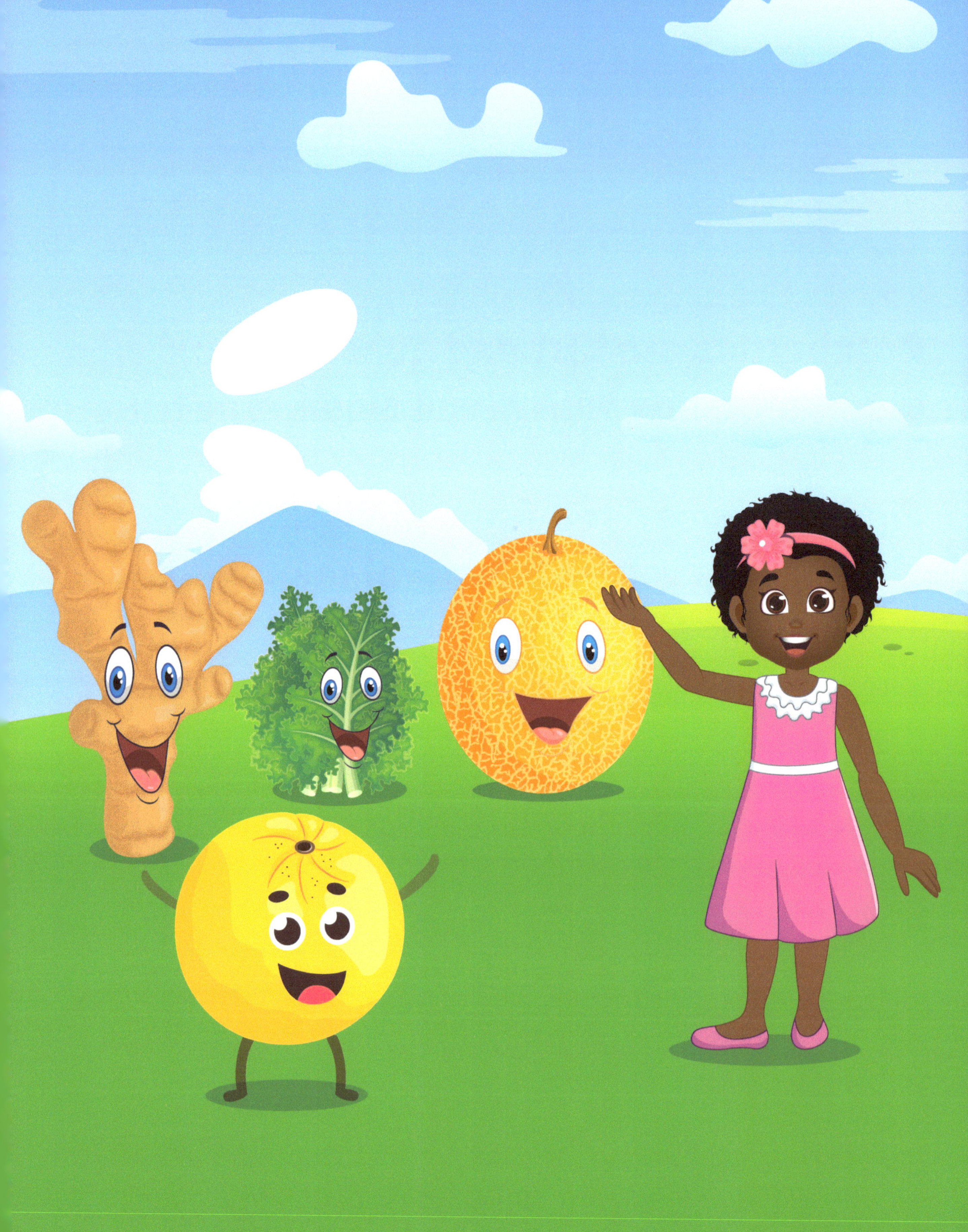

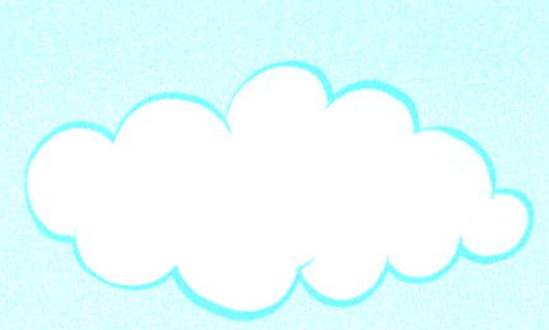

Ginger adds flavor with a spicy slice,
grapefruit's sour taste is quite precise.

Honeydew is sweet and full of bliss,
kale helps your vision, so you never miss.

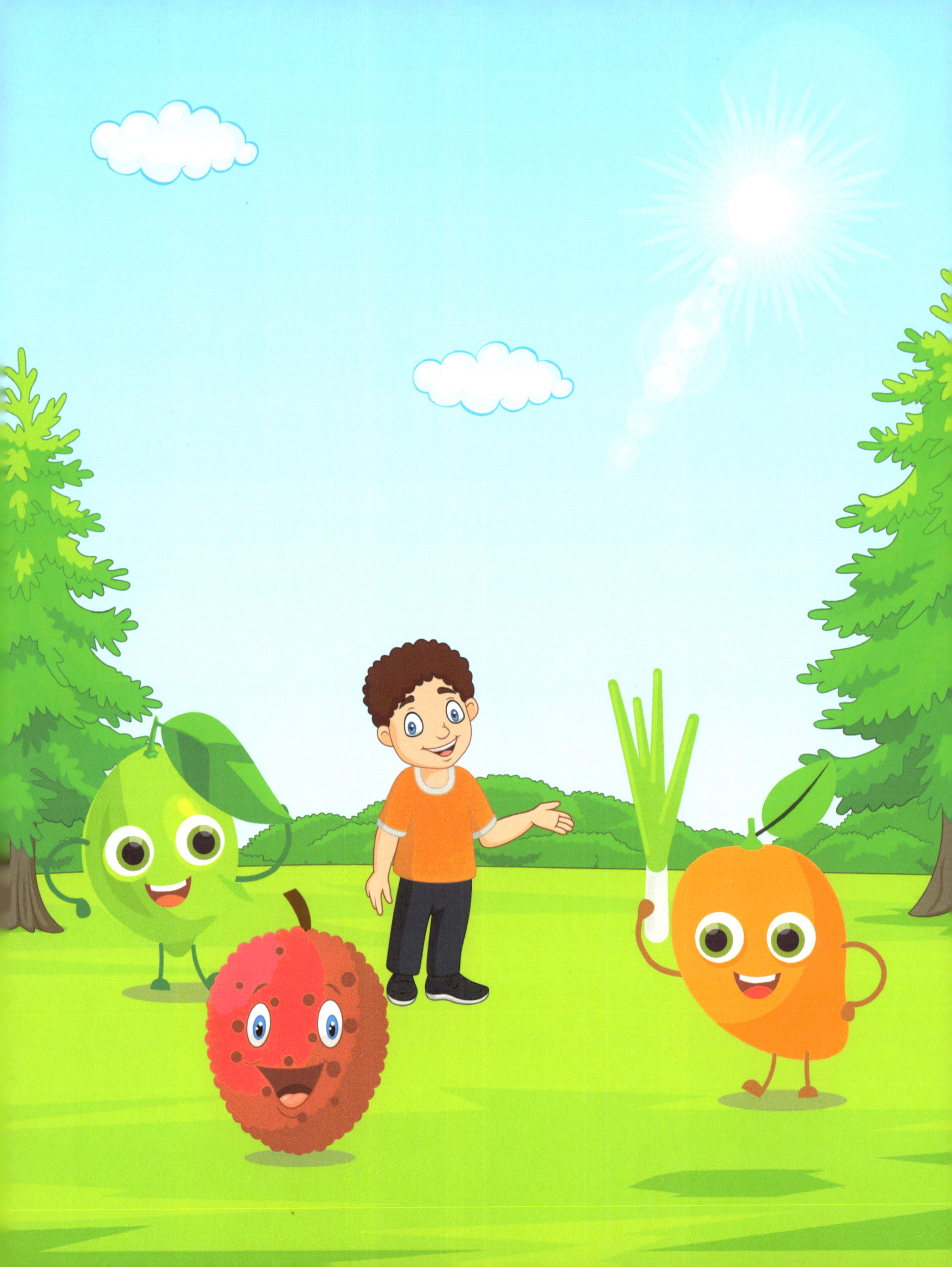

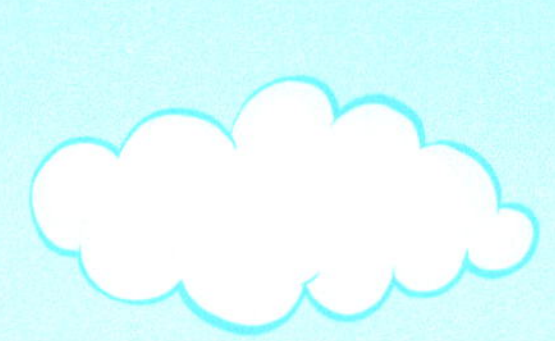

Leeks help you feel good through and through, lime adds zest to your food, it's true.

Lychee is sweet like a sunny day, mangoes keep you healthy, come what may.

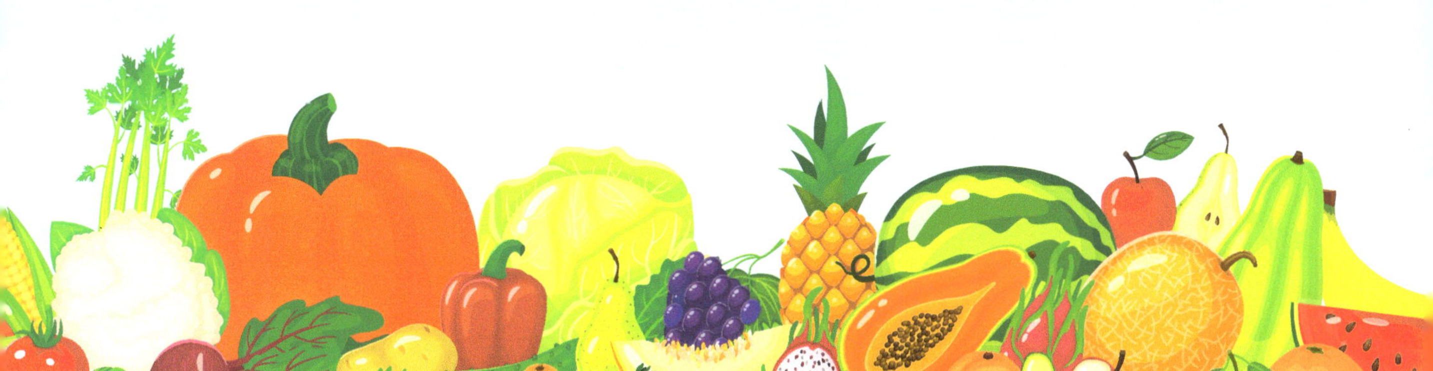

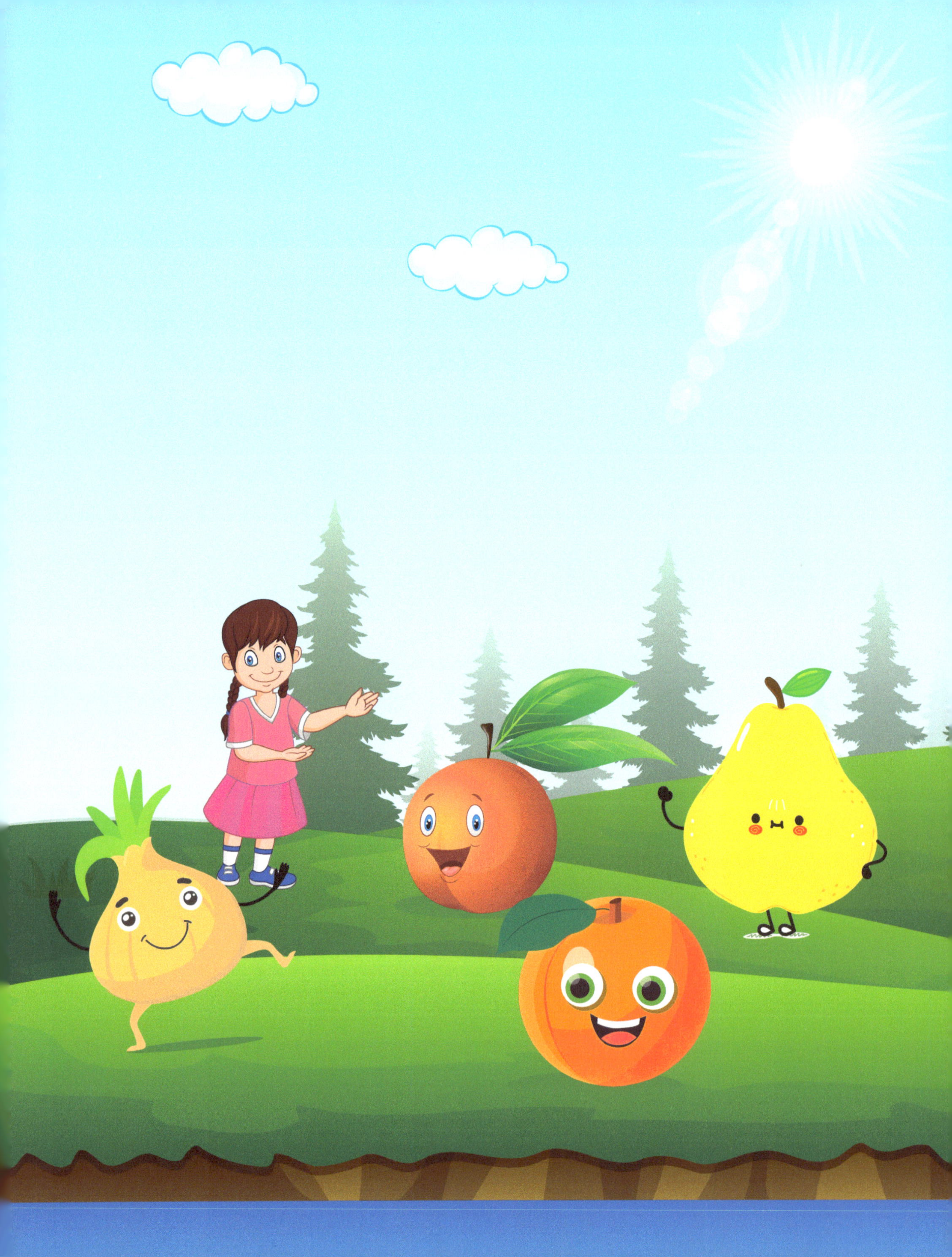

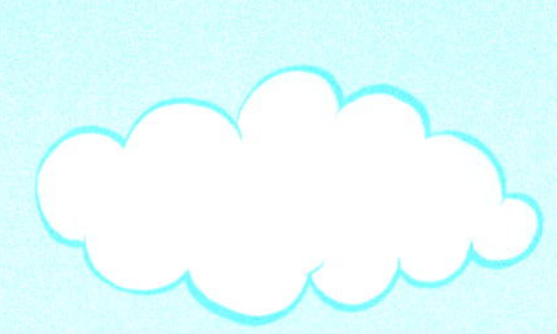

Nectarines keep you feeling fresh,
onions help your heart stay its best.

Peaches are sweet and oh so divine,
pears help your digestion, so you feel just fine.

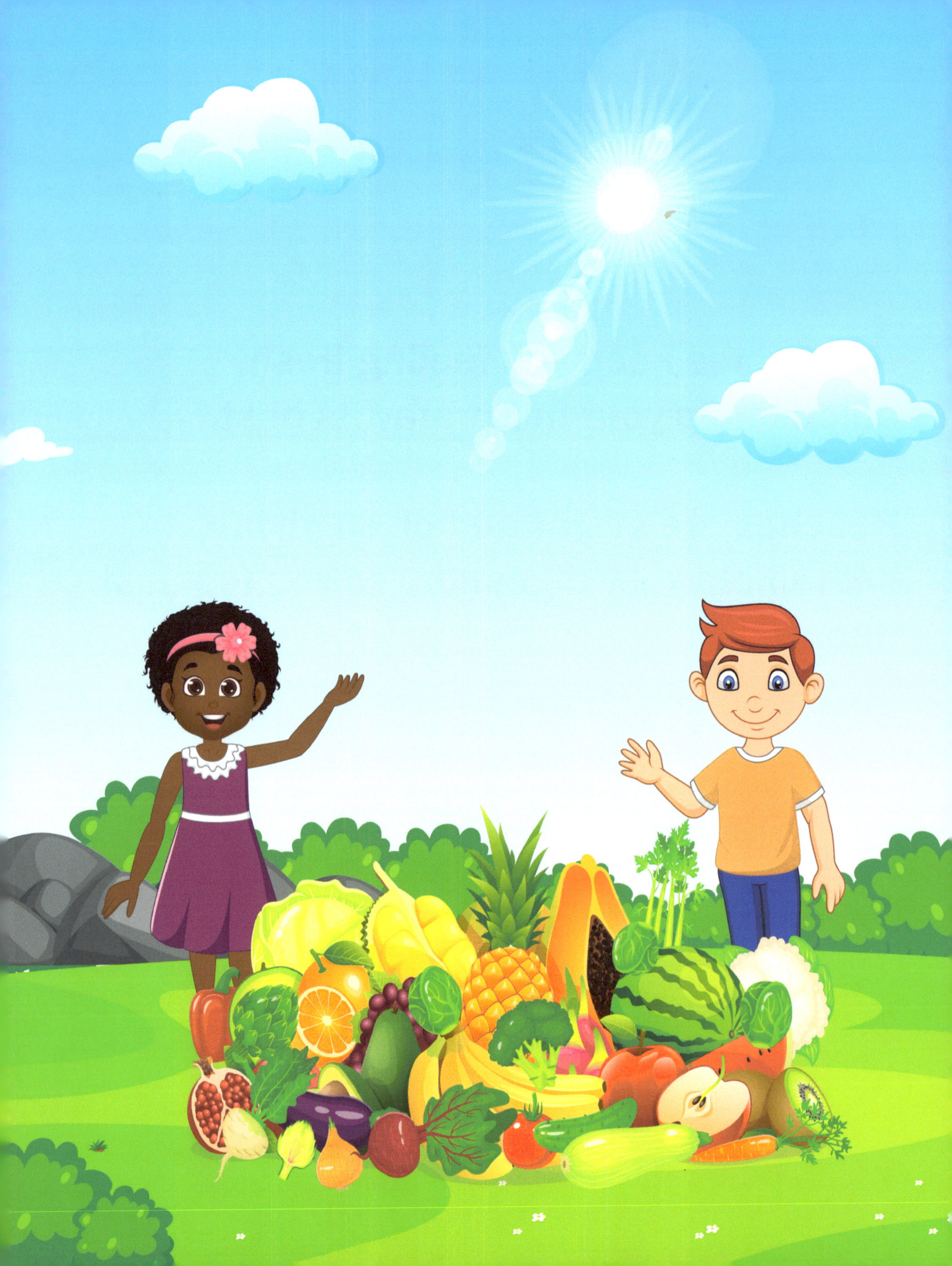

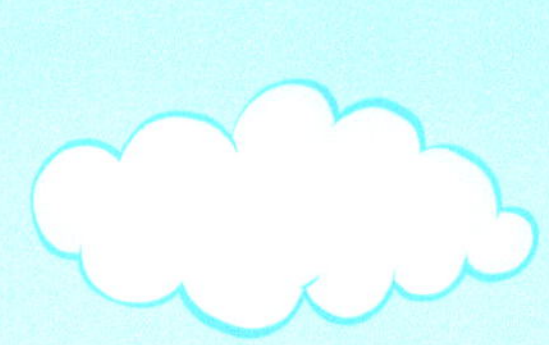

So eat your fruits and veggies each day,
They'll keep you healthy in every way!

Your body will thank you, just wait and see
and you'll feel strong, healthy, and happy
as can be!